ICS 11.040.99

**SCM-C**

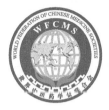

世界中医药学会联合会
**World Federation of Chinese Medicine Societies**

**SCM-C 0039-2020**

# 温控红外灸疗垫

## Thermo-controlled Infrared Moxibustion-like Pad

U0306119

世界中联分支机构标准
**Committee Standard of WFCMS**

2020–01–17发布实施
**Issued and implemented on Jan. 17th, 2020**

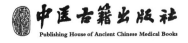

中医古籍出版社
Publishing House of Ancient Chinese Medical Books

**图书在版编目（CIP）数据**

温控红外灸疗垫：汉英对照 / 世界中医药学会联合
会著 . —北京：中医古籍出版社，2020.10

ISBN 978-7-5152-2041-3

Ⅰ.①温… Ⅱ.①世… Ⅲ.①艾灸—医疗器械—汉、
英 Ⅳ.① R245.81 ② TH772

中国版本图书馆 CIP 数据核字（2020）第 134162 号

**温控红外灸疗垫**

世界中医药学会联合会　著

责任编辑　王晓曼
特约编辑　张　楚
出版发行　中医古籍出版社
社　　址　北京东直门内南小街 16 号（100700）
电　　话　010-64089446（总编室）010-64002949（发行部）
网　　址　www.zhongyiguji.com.cn
印　　刷　北京建宏印刷有限公司
开　　本　880mm×1230mm　1/16
印　　张　1.25
字　　数　39 千字
版　　次　2020 年 10 月第 1 版　2020 年 10 月第 1 次印刷
书　　号　ISBN 978-7-5152-2041-3
定　　价　36.00 元

# 目　次

# 前　言

请注意本标准的某些内容可能涉及专利。本标准的发布机构不承担识别这些专利的责任。

**本标准的主要起草单位：**嘉兴福气多温控床有限公司、珠海市元生健商贸有限公司、嘉善臻成健身器材厂、上海中医药大学、天津中医药大学、芜湖圣美孚科技有限公司、无锡佳健医疗器械股份有限公司。

**本标准主要起草人：**

中　　国：曲雅芝、林东岳、申玉柳、于志学、苏运东、曲玉成、张怀鹏、于志峰、王联、王文清、杨华元

泰　　国：Tamar Buranatawonsom

澳大利亚：Jack Zheng

本标准的起草程序遵守了世界中医药学会联合会发布的 SCM 0001-2009《标准制定和发布工作规范》和世界中医药学会联合会秘书处发布的世界中联秘发 2011（20 号）文件《世界中联各专业委员会专业技术标准制定实施办法》。

本标准由世界中医药学会联合会中医诊疗仪器专业委员会发布，版权归世界中医药学会联合会所有。

# 温控红外灸疗垫

## 1 范围

本文件规定了温控红外灸疗垫的术语、规格与型号、技术要求、检验方法、检验规则及标志、包装、运输、贮存。

本文件适用于不可洗涤的温控红外灸疗垫。

## 2 规范性引用文件

下列文件对于本文件的应用必不可少。凡是标注日期的引用文件，仅标注日期的版本适用于本文件。凡是不标注日期的引用文件，其最新版本（包括所有的修改单）适用于本文件。

ISO 20493:2018 *Infrared moxibusition-like instruments*

IEC 60601–1–2:2014 *Medical electrical equipment— Part 1-2: General requirements for basic safety and essential performance—Collateral standard: Electromagnetic disturbances-Requirements and tests*

IEC 60601–1–11:2015 *Medical electrical equipment— Part 1-11: General requirements for basic safety and essential performance— Collateral standard: Requirements for medical electrical equipment and medical electrical systems used in the home healthcare environment*

ISO 780:2015 *Packaging-Distribution packaging-Graphical symbols for handling and storage of packages*

ISO/IEC Guide 37:2012 *Instructions for use of products by consumers*

GB 4343.2-2009 家用电器、电动工具和类似器具的电磁兼容要求 第 2 部分：抗扰度

GB 4706.1-2005 家电和类似用途电器的安全 第一部分：通用要求

GB 4706.8-2008 家用和类似用途电器的安全 电热毯、电热垫及类似柔性发热器具的特殊要求

GB/T 4654-2008 非金属基体红外辐射加热器通用技术条件

GB/T 7287-2008 红外辐射加热器试验方法

## 3 术语和定义

下列术语和定义适用于本文件。

### 3.1 正常工作

输入交流电压 220V，垫处于平铺，无折叠且上表面放有一定的覆盖物（被子、人体）的状态。

### 3.2 发热元件

以硅胶电热丝、无磁界电热丝、带屏蔽的电热丝等组成具有发热作用的元件。

### 3.3 柔性部件

以发热元件和所有其他辅助材料构成的器具或可拆卸的外罩。

### 3.4 温控红外灸疗垫

一种通过加热到一定程度，产生 1 ～ 10μm 范围红外辐射波长，具有灸疗效应的垫。

注：温控红外灸疗垫包括颈椎垫、腰椎垫、床垫。

## 4 规格与型号命名

### 4.1 规格

温控红外灸疗垫的规格应符合表 1 的规定。

表 1　各类产品规格

| 品种 | 尺寸（mm） | | 厚度 |
|---|---|---|---|
| | 长度 | 宽度 | |
| 单人床垫 | 1900、2000、2030、1500 | 1000、1200、550 | 厚度 ≥ 50 |
| 双人床垫 | 1900、2000、2030 | 1350、1500、1530 | |
| | 2000 | 1800 | |
| 颈椎垫 | 450、420、410、400、390、350 | 330、300、210、190、140 | |
| 腰椎垫 | 1280、900、700、550 | 550、460、450、350 | |
| 允差 | ±5 | | |

### 4.2 型号命名

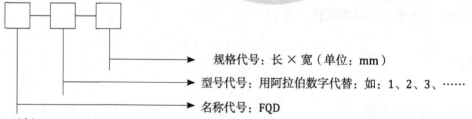

规格代号：长 × 宽（单位：mm）

型号代号：用阿拉伯数字代替：如：1、2、3、……

名称代号：FQD

示例：FQD-1（1900mm×1500mm）表示为：型号为 FQD-1 型规格为 1900mm×1500mm 的红外灸疗床垫

## 5 技术要求

### 5.1 外观

表面应平整，不能有任何损坏现象。

### 5.2 温度控制

5.2.1 在规定的试验条件下，温升不小于17K，产品表面最高平均温度不高于45℃。

5.2.2 控制温度误差不大于±5℃。

5.2.3 产品可调温度为20～60℃，具有12小时自动断电功能。

### 5.3 无线电干扰和电视干扰的抑制

具有屏蔽有害电磁波的功能，应符合GB 4343.2-2009规定。

### 5.4 电器安全性

电气安全通用要求应符合IEC 60601-1-11:2015的规定。

### 5.5 远红外线发射率

远红外线发射率≥0.83。

### 5.6 红外辐射波长范围（μm）

产品在受热时可产生波长为1～10μm的远红外线的发热区域。

## 6 测试方法

### 6.1 温升

按照GB 4706.1-2005标准中的要求规定进行测试，其结果应符合5.2的要求。

### 6.2 无线电干扰和电视干扰的抑制

按照GB 4343.2-2009规定进行测试，其结果应符合5.3的要求。

### 6.3 电器安全性

按照IEC 60601-1-11:2015、IEC 60601-1-2:2014规定的方法进行试验；其结果应符合5.4的要求。

### 6.4 额定功率

用电参数测试仪进行测试。

## 6.5 远红外线发射率

按照 GB/T 4654-2008，GB/T 7287-2008 标准中相关条款进行测试，其结果应符合 5.5 的要求。

## 6.6 红外辐射波长范围

按照 GB/T 4654-2008，GB/T 7287-2008 标准中相关条款进行测试，其结果应符合 5.6 的要求。

# 7 检验规则

## 7.1 检验分类

检验分为出厂检验和型式检验。

## 7.2 出厂检验

7.2.1 产品由制造厂质量检验部门检验合格后并附合格证方可出厂。

7.2.2 出厂检验为逐一检验，制造商应在注册产品标准中规定出厂检验项目。出厂检验的结果判定分为合格与不合格两种，检验不合格者可修正后再进行检验。

## 7.3 型式试验

7.3.1 型式试验是本标准的所有技术要求。

7.3.2 型式试验在正常生产情况下，每年检验一次。发生下列情况之一时也应进行型式试验：

a）产品转厂生产的试制定型鉴定；

b）产品停产半年以上重新生产时；

c）当设计、工艺、材料有重大改变时；

d）当出现质量事故或重大质量波动时；

e）国家质量监督机构提出进行型式检验要求时。

## 7.3.3 型式检验的样品

从出厂检验合格产品中随机抽取 1 台。

## 7.3.4 型式检验检测的项目

所有检验项目全部合格，则判定型式检测合格。型式检验未通过时，不得进行批量生产。

# 8 标志、标签、使用说明书、包装、运输和贮存

## 8.1 标志

8.1.1 标志应符合 ISO 15223-1 的要求。

8.1.2 产品至少应有下列外部标志：

a）制造厂名称和商标；

b）产品名称和型号；

c）电源电压；

d）电源频率；

e）输入功率；

f）产品注册编号。

8.1.3 外包装箱上至少应有下列标志：

a）制造厂名称；

b）制造厂地址；

c）产品名称和型号；

d）毛重、净重；

e）体积；

f）数量；

g）生产日期；

h）产品注册号；

i）产品标准号；

j）箱体上的字样和标志应保证不因历时较久而模糊不清。

## 8.2 标签

检验合格证上应有下列内容：

a）制造厂名称；

b）产品名称；

c）检验日期；

d）检验员代号。

## 8.3 使用说明书

使用说明书应有下列主要内容：

a）主要性能指标；

b）适用范围；

c）储运条件；

d）安装要求；

e）使用方法及注意事项；

f）安全使用规则；

g）常见故障排除；

h）维护及保养；

i）警告语；

j）售后服务承诺。

## 8.4 包装

8.4.1 包装应有可靠的防潮、防尘措施，保证产品的绝缘性和保护层不受损伤。

8.4.2 出厂产品应包括完整的产品、使用说明书、产品合格证、产品保修卡等。

8.4.3 包装箱标记应包括制造厂全名、产品名称、产品型号、产品规格；按规定程序办理的商标、产品数量、收货单位名称和地址、包装箱外形尺寸、注意事项标志"小心轻放、切勿受潮"等文字或符号、出厂日期等。

## 8.5 运输

运输方式由制造商与客户商定。产品在运输过程中应有遮盖物和进行的必要的防护，防止局部重压和雨淋。

## 8.6 贮存

产品应贮存在干燥、通风良好的仓库中，贮存环境温度应为 –10 ～ 40℃，相对湿度不超过80%，确保无腐蚀性气体。

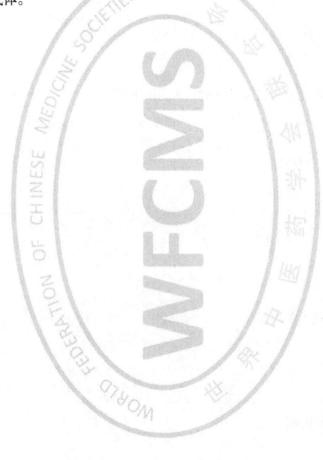

# Preface

Attention is drawn to the possibility that some of the elements of this standard may be the subject of patent rights. The issuing body of this document shall not be held responsible for identifying any or all such patent rights.

Main Drafting Units of this standard: Jiaxing Fuqiduo Temperature Control Instrument Co., Ltd., Zhuhai Yuanshengjian Trading Co., Ltd., Jiashan Zhencheng Fitness Equipment Co., Ltd., Shanghai University of Traditional Chinese Medicine, Tianjin University of Traditional Chinese Medicine, Wuhu Saint Mobil Technology Co., Ltd., Wuxi Jiajian Medical Instrument Co., Ltd.

Drafters and reviewers of this standard:

**China:** Qu Yazhi, Lin Dongyue, Shen Yuliu, Yu Zhixue, Su Yundong, Qu Yucheng, Zhang Huaipeng, Yu Zhifeng, Wang Lian, Wang Wenqing, Yang Huayuan.

**Thailand:** Tamar Buranatawonsom.

**Austrilia:** Jack Zheng.

The drafting procedures of this standard were consistent with *SCM 0001-2009 Working Regulation for Formulation and Publication of Standard* and document of *2011 (No. 20) Implementation of Technical Standards of the Specialized Committee* released by World Federation of Chinese Medicine Societies (WFCMS).

All copyrights are reserved to WFCMS.

# Thermo-controlled infrared moxibustion-like pad

## 1  Scope

This standard specifies the terms and definitions, specifications and models, technical requirements, inspection methods and rules, and signs, packaging, transportation and storage of thermo-controlled infrared moxibustion-like pad.

This standard is applicable to the non-washed thermo-controlled infrared moxibustion-like pad.

## 2  Normative references

The following documents are referred to in the text in such a way that some or all of their content constitutes requirements of this document. For dated references, only the edition cited applies. For undated references, the latest edition of the referenced document (including any amendments) applies.

ISO 20493:2018  *Infrared moxibusition-like instruments*

IEC 60601-1-2:2014  *Medical electrical equipment — Part 1-2: General requirements for basic safety and essential performance—Collateral standard: Electromagnetic disturbances-Requirements and tests*

IEC 60601-1-11:2015  *Medical electrical equipment — Part 1-11: General requirements for basic safety and essential performance — Collateral standard: Requirements for medical electrical equipment and medical electrical systems used in the home healthcare environment*

ISO 780:2015  *Packaging-Distribution packaging-Graphical symbols for handling and storage of packages*

ISO/IEC Guide 37:2012  *Instructions for use of products by consumers*

GB 4343.2-2009  *Electromagnetic compatibility requirements for household appliances, power tools and similar appliances  Part 2: immunity from disturbance*

GB 4706.1-2005  *Safety of electrical appliances and similar apparatus  Part 1: General requirements*

GB 4706.8-2008  *Safety of electrical appliances and similar apparatus   Special requirements for electric blankets, electric pads and similar flexible heating apparatus.*

GB/T 4654-2008  *General specification for non-metallic matrix infrared radiation heaters*

GB/T 7287-2008  *Test method for infrared radiation heater*

## 3  Terms and definitions

For the purposes of this document, the following terms and definitions apply.

### 3.1 Regular work

A state that inputting AC voltage 220 V, pad is tiling, no folding, and with a certain covering (quilt or human body) put on it.

### 3.2 Heating element

An element composed of silica gel electric heating wire, non-magnetic boundary electric heating wire, shielded electric heating wire, etc.

### 3.3 Flexible component

An apparatus or detachable enclosure made of heating elements and all other auxiliary materials.

### 3.4 Thermo-controlled infrared moxibustion-like pad

A kind of pat that can produce infrared radiation wavelength in the range of 1~10 μm by heating to a certain extent with the similar effect of moxibustion therapy.

Note: Thermo-controlled infrared moxibustion-like pads include cervical spine pad, lumbar pad, and mattress.

## 4 Specifications and models nomenclature

### 4.1 Specifications

The specifications of thermo-controlled infrared moxibustion-like pads shall comply with the provisions of Table 1.

Table 1. Product specifications

| Types | Size (mm) | | Thickness |
|---|---|---|---|
| | Length | Width | |
| Single-bed mattress | 1900, 2000, 2030, 1500 | 1000, 1200, 550 | Thickness ≥ 50 |
| Twin-bed mattress | 1900, 2000, 2030 | 1350, 1500, 1530 | |
| | 2000 | 1800 | |
| Cervical spine pad | 450, 420, 410, 400, 390, 350 | 330, 300, 210, 190, 140 | |
| Lumbar pad | 1280, 900, 700, 550 | 550, 460, 450, 350 | |
| Tolerance | ±5 | | |

## 4.2 Models nomenclature

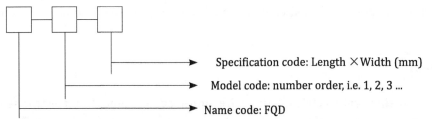

Specification code: Length ×Width (mm)

Model code: number order, i.e. 1, 2, 3 ...

Name code: FQD

Example:FQD-1 (1900mm×1500mm) is for the thermo-controlled infrared moxibustion-like pad of the type of FQD-1, with the size of 1900mm×1500mm.

## 5  Technical requirements

### 5.1  Appearance

The surface shall be flat without any damage.

### 5.2  Temperature control

**5.2.1**   The temperature rise is no less than 17K and the maximum average temperature of the product surface is no more than 45°C, under specified test conditions.

**5.2.2**   The error in temperature control shall be no more than ±5°C.

**5.2.3**   The adjustable temperature of the product is 20~60°C and it has 12-hour automatic power-off function.

### 5.3  Shield against radio and television signal interference

The products have the function of shielding harmful electromagnetic waves and shall comply with GB 4343.2-2009.

### 5.4  Electrical safeties

General requirements for electrical safeties shall comply with IEC 60601-1-11:2015.

### 5.5  Remote infrared emissivity

Remote infrared emissivity shall be no less than 0.83.

### 5.6  Range of infrared radiation wavelength (μm)

The product can form a heating area with remote infrared ray with a wavelength of 1μm to 10μm when heated.

## 6 Test methods

### 6.1 Temperature rise

The test shall be in accordance with the requirements in GB 4706.1-2005 and the test results shall meet the requirements of 5.2 in GB 4706.1-2005.

### 6.2 Shield of radio interference and television interference

The test shall be in accordance with the requirements in GB 4343.2-2009 and the test results shall meet the requirements of 5.3 in GB 4343.2-2009.

### 6.3 Electrical safeties

The test shall be in accordance with the requirements in IEC 60601-1-11:2015 and IEC 60601-1-2:2014 and the test results shall meet the corresponding requirements.

### 6.4 Rated power

Rated power shall be tested by electrical parameters tester.

### 6.5 Remote infrared emissivity

The test shall be in accordance with the requirements in GB/T 4654-2008 and GB/T 7287-2008 and the test results shall meet the corresponding requirements in 5.5.

### 6.6 Range of infrared radiation wavelength

The test shall be in accordance with the requirements in GB/T 4654-2008 and GB/T 7287-2008 and the test results shall meet the corresponding requirements in 5.6.

## 7 Verification norm

### 7.1 Classification

It is divided into outgoing quality control test and type test.

### 7.2 Outgoing quality control test

**7.2.1** The products shall be inspected by the quality control department of the manufacturer and only with a certificate of conformity can the qualified products leave the factory.

**7.2.2** The product shall be tested one by one during the outgoing quality control test and the manufacturer shall specify the test items in the corresponding standard of registered product. The results of the test includes two type, qualified and unqualified. The unqualified products shall retest after reparation.

### 7.3 Type test

**7.3.1** Type test includes all the technical requirements of this standard.

**7.3.2** The type test is normally conducted once a year under normal conditions. Type tests shall be carried out in any of the following cases:

a) when trial production finalization for product produced in other factory;

b) when the production is discontinued for over half a year;

c) when there are major changes in design, process and materials;

d) when there is a quality accident or a major quality fluctuation;

e) When the quality supervision agency of the different nations requests type test.

### 7.3.3 Type test sample

The sample shall be randomly selected from the qualified products after outgoing quality control test.

### 7.3.4 Items in type test

If the product is qualified all items, then it is qualified in the type test. Mass production shall not be carried out if the type test fails.

## 8 Sign, label, instructions, packaging, transportation and storage

### 8.1 Sign

**8.1.1** Sign shall be in accordance with the requirements in ISO 15223-1.

**8.1.2** The products shall have at least the following signs:

a) Manufacturer's name and trademark;

b) Product name and model;

c) Supply voltage;

d) Power frequency;

e) Input power;

f) Product registration number.

**8.1.3** The external package shall include at least the following signs:

a) Manufacturer's name;

b) Manufacturer's address;

c) Product name and model;

d)Gross and net weight;

e) Size;

f) Quantity;

g) Manufacturing Date;

h) Product registration number;

i) Product standard number;

j) The words and signs on the box shall not be blurred during a period of time.

## 8.2   Label

The product qualification label shall include the following information:

a) Manufacturer's name;

b) Product name;

c) Test date;

d) Tester's code.

## 8.3   Instructions

Instructions shall include the following information:

a) Main performance figures;

b) Application scope;

c) Storage and transportation conditions;

d) Installing requirement;

e) Usage and Precautions;

f) Rules of safety use;

g) Troubleshooting;

h) Maintenance;

i) Warnings;

j) After-sales service commitment.

## 8.4   Packaging

**8.4.1**   Packaging shall have reliable moisture-proof and dust-proof measures to ensure the insulation and protection of the layer of products.

**8.4.2**   The outgoing products shall include complete products, instructions, product qualification label, warranty card, etc.

**8.4.3**   The packages shall include the manufacturer's full name, product name, product model, product specification, trademark, product quantity, name and address of the retailer, packing box shape and size, signs and labels including " Handle with care" or " abstaining from moistness", date of departure, etc.

## 8.5   Transportation

The transport mode is agreed upon by the manufacturer and the customer. Covering and necessary protection during transportation is to prevent heavy pressure in certain parts and rains.

## 8.6   Storage

The product shall be stored in a dry, well-ventilated warehouse, with the environment temperature of -10~40°C and the relative humidity of no more than 80%, and without corrosive gas.